Book Of The Best Mouth Care

Procedure

Olatundun Solomon

olatundunsolomon@gmail.com

goodhealth1234567.blogspot. com

I have Honor Code Certificate from the University of Texas System edx. The course is 4.01x: Take Your Medicine-The Impact of Drug Development.

Am a Certified Alison Graduate with distinction in the course: Diploma in Nursing and Patient Care.

I have Honor Code Certificate from Harvard University through edx in the course PH201x: Health and Society.

Am a Certified Alison Graduate with distinction in the course: Diploma in Human Nutrition.

I also have Honor Code Certificate from edx Karolinska Institutet in the course KIBEHMEDx: Behavioral Medicine: A Key to Better Health.

Mouth

The mouth is the part of the body that comprises of the lips, tongue, teeth, the palate and also the mouth cavity.

Saliva is normally present in the mouth. This is produced from the salivary glands. The salivary glands are parotid gland, sublingual gland and submandibular gland. The saliva makes food that is placed in the mouth to be wet and this makes the food to be easily chewed. The saliva also makes the digestion of carbohydrate food to occur, because there is amylase in it, cause digestion of carbohydrate to happen in the mouth. Saliva makes the chewed food to be swallowed comfortably and it passes the throat easily. The teeth is used to cut and chew food. It makes digestion to occur easily by increasing the surface area for the digestion of food. This prevents choking effect of food when it is swallowed. The teeth

when it is white indicates cleanliness

of it. And it shows the absence of

pathogens (disease causing

microorganisms). It also indicates

the absence of tooth caries (tooth

decay).

The gums in the mouth, when it is

not bleeding and when there is no

inflammation indicates healthy gums.

When the palate is not cleft palate,

and it is clean and is not inflamed or

bleeds it shows that it is free from infection.

The mouth is very important to be taken care of. This makes it to be healthy.

The tongue that is used for taste, for speech and also for eating needs to be healthy, in order to carry out its functions effectively. The tongue can test sour food. It can also test bitter food. It can test sweet food and salty food. When there is inflammation of the tongue (glossitis) due to infection, vitamin deficiency and

also anaemia. This can be prevented

by eating balanced diet

(carbohydrate, protein, unsaturated

fatty acid from vegetable oil,

minerals, vitamins, and water) and

having oral hygiene.

The teeth, tongue, gums and also

the palate needs proper care. When

this is done, it prevents bad

breath(halitosis). It makes bacteria

not to be

Mouth	Teeth	Lips	Palate	Tongue	Gums

parts are:					

present in the mouth. It do not make

infection to be transferred from

husband to wife or from wife to

husband when they kiss. All the

human body needs to be well taken

care of, because disease can be

transferred from a part of the

human body to another part. For

example, malignant cancer can

metastasize from the nose into the

mouth.

It is good to go to the hospital for regular check up.

The mouth of children, adults, old age people and people that are ill needs proper care.

Mouth hygiene makes the person to eat and swallow food without pain. It also makes the person to speak well because of the absence of tooth decay and gum disease.

The extension of infection from the mouth to other part of the body is not actualized because there is

mouth hygiene.

Teeth: the teeth has the crown and

the root. There is canine, incisors,

premolar and molar type of teeth.

The crown is the normal whitish part

that can be seen when the mouth is

opened. The root is inside the gum.

The teeth is very hard and strong.

It is used for cutting and chewing

food. This makes the food to be

ready for swallowing after it as been mixed with saliva.

The teeth can be removed by using an object that is hard to hit it with a big force, this should be prevented.

Tooth infection such as tooth decay and cavitation can occur. This happens when the teeth is not properly taken care of.

Pus can be seen in the surface of the gums when there is infection of the teeth that progress to the gums.

Food that contain sucrose, when present on the teeth it is fermented by bacteria. This results to plaque formation on the teeth, and the acid that is formed demineralize the bone by causing cavity. This is because, calcium and phosphorus in the teeth is reduced. For example, eating sweet cake at night before going to bed and not brushing the teeth with toothpaste and toothbrush. There will be fragments of the food in the mouth. Bacteria will ferment the remnant sweet cake in the mouth into acid by making it

to become plaque on the teeth

(tooth caries). This will cause

demineralization of the teeth(teeth

break down). This will lead to cavity

formation in the teeth. This will also

result to tooth pain(odontodynia).

Infection can cause inflammation of

the gums(gingivitis). This makes the

person to not be comfortable. This is

because of the swollen gums, it is

reddish, there is heat and pain. If

this is not prevented other teeth can

be affected, leading to the same results. This can eventually cause tooth loose. Other food fragments in the mouth that is not washed away by cleaning the mouth can also cause it to occur.

Vomiting(emesis) of food from the stomach can cause it. This is because the stomach as gastric acid. When the mouth is not washed properly with water after vomiting, it makes acidic contents in the mouth to demineralize the teeth. Thereby making the teeth to breakdown and have plaque on it. Which will make the teeth to have cavity in it. The teeth will not be able to be used for chewing food because of the cavity, pain, heat, redness of the gums and swollen gums.

Eating of unwashed fruits can cause teeth infections from the microorganisms that is present on the fruits.

Also eating food that is not well cooked can cause it, because microorganisms may be present that may act in that undercooked food and may cause infection to the teeth.

Using of very hard brush can wear the teeth, thereby causing demineralization to the teeth. Using the teeth to open the metal cork cover can cause demineralization to the teeth.

Using the teeth by children to hold ropes can make another child to hold the other end of it and pulling it. It can make the teeth to be removed.

Punch on the mouth can remove the teeth.

Using tetracycline as drug by little children can cause teeth discoloration. Using drugs for teeth care without consulting medical doctors in the hospital can causing adverse effect to the teeth. It can lead to other organs of the body to be affected adversely.

By not making sure the toothbrush is kept clean can cause infection to the teeth. Other diseases that may be in the body should be treated before pregnancy.

Prenatal(before the birth of a child that is in the womb), natal(during the period of the birth of a child), perinatal(during the time of birth), and post natal(after birth) care should be done in the hospital.

Milk is good for the teeth to grow. It contains calcium and phosphate that is good for healthy teeth growth. Fish, vegetables and egg are also good for teeth growth.

After the birth of the child by a

pregnant woman. She should feed

the child with breast milk by breast

feeding the child. All the nutrients

the child needs are in the breast milk.

When the mouth is injured eating

food such as pepper, garlic, ginger

and other spices may be very

uncomfortable. Treatment should be

done effectively in the hospital.

Then the person can eat spicy food.

Care Of The Teeth In Order To

Prevent Diseases

Toothbrushing: This is a method that should be used to take good care of the teeth. The teeth should be brushed in the morning after breakfast and after dinner.

When the teeth is having part that is yellowish and black, this is sign of tooth decay. When there is tooth decay and tooth cavitation, the person is uncomfortable to speak, sleep, to eat, and to express his or her feelings. It is good to prevent

this by cleaning the teeth and the

mouth as a whole, in order to

prevent infection.

It is good to brush with a small head

tooth brush that is soft in order to

prevent trauma(injury) to the gums

and also prevent wearing of teeth.

When brush with very hard bristle is

used, it may lead to easy erosion of

the teeth. This can lead to pain of

the teeth that can make cutting and

chewing of food to be

uncomfortable. This method removes remnant of food particles that may be in the mouth after eating in the morning and at night. When food remnants that are in the mouth are not properly removed it can cause bacteria to ferment it and it will cause acid to be formed by causing demineralization of teeth. This will cause tooth caries and cavitation of the teeth.

It is good to use toothpaste that has fluoride, it prevent tooth caries. The toothbrush should be washed and kept clean after use.

When a very big brush is used, it can easily cause gum trauma(injury) and the bleeding of gums.

The toothbrush head should be small and the bristles should be soft. This prevents gum injury and makes the toothbrush to be able to touch different corners of the teeth, in order to clean it and to make it healthy.

Toothbrush and toothpaste that as fluoride in it should be used. The fluoride prevents tooth caries.

After washing the teeth with the toothbrush and toothpaste the mouth should be properly rinsed with water and the water should be poured out from the mouth. The mouth should be gargled with water and it should be poured out. This do not make food particles to be present in the mouth. Thereby preventing tooth decay to be formed.

This also prevents bad

breath(halitosis).

Tooth scaling is also implored, by

using different instruments to

remove food particles in the mouth

that is left after eating.

Electric toothbrush is also good to be

used. It is very effective by using

electric current supply power to the

toothbrush. This makes

toothbrushing to be easy and

efficient. Plaques are prevented

from forming on the teeth. This

makes the teeth not to demineralize,

but cause the teeth to remineralize.

Flossing can also be done by a dental

hygienist. Flossing makes different

parts of the body to be properly

clean, by removing plaques from it.

Different corners of the teeth is

made clean and healthy. After the

removal of calculi(plaque), acid

formation is not present. This

prevents cavitation of the teeth as a

result of demineralization. This is

because of good oral hygiene.

Interdental brush can be used also to keep the teeth clean. Normal size should be used to prevent, too large or too small size. In order to prevent injury to the gums and wearing of the teeth. The interdental brush should brush between teeth to keep it healthy. After that, the mouth should be gargled with water and it should be poured out. After the interdental brush as been used, it should be washed with soup and rinsed with water and kept clean. Another interdental brush should be purchased after bristles of the it have reduced due to wear and tear.

Tongue scrapers is effective in the removal microorganisms from the tongue surface. This is achieved by using it to scrape the surfaces of the tongue to keep it clean and healthy. After which the mouth is gargled with water and poured out from the mouth. This prevents contagious diseases through kissing from husband to wife or from the wife to the husband. This also prevent communicable diseases through coughing.

Washing of the hand frequently is also good in order to prevent contagious diseases.

Washing of the rugs, cleaning the tiles, washing of the clothes, cleaning the shoes, cleaning the chairs, doing environmental sanitation around the house and cleaning up the house as a whole prevents infections.

Oral irrigation is good to be done to keep the mouth clean. Sublingual irrigation is the irrigation of under the tongue. This makes under the tongue to be free from pathogens(disease causing microorganisms). And this prevents halitosis (bad breath).

Single tufted brushes are also useful to be used for hygienic teeth and tongue. It makes it possible to brush nooks and crannies of the teeth. Makes plaques to be prevented from affecting the teeth. Therefore, demineralization of the teeth does not occur. Massaging of the gums can be done by using gum stimulators in order to make good blood circulation to happen. This results to an healthy gums that is well nourished. This prevents the gums from fatigue.

When there is less blood supply to the teeth it cause pains to the gums(gingivalgia). Because the gum is less nourished by the nutrients in the blood, due to low blood supply.

It also makes injury to the gums to

not heal quickly due to less fibrin

supply.

Gingivitis (inflammation of the gums)

should be prevented by not drinking

dirty water that can cause infection

to the teeth that can result to it.

Good oral(mouth) hygiene is good to

keep the mouth clean.

In the hospital efficient mouth

washing can be done to keep the

tongue very clean, the teeth very

whitish and the mouth as a whole to be very clean. In the hospital there can be diagnosis through blood test, MRI scanning and X-ray scanning. And preventive measures can be made. In the hospital the use of antibiotics, disinfectants and antibacterial drugs may be prescribed. In order for the body to be free from pathogens(disease causing microorganisms). It is good to follow the drug prescription by the medical doctor in order to prevent diseases of the mouth.

Eating of food that contain spices are good to prevent infections. This makes the mouth to be free from infections, that can cause gingivopathy(gums diseases). e.g. gingivitis (inflammation of the gums). This also prevents pathogens (diseases causing microorganisms), from the gums to other parts of the body.

Eating soup that has green vegetables is good for the production of blood. This makes the mouth to be healthy. The gums is

well nourished because of much

blood supply to the gums. This cause

the gums to be healthy and free

from fatigue.

Eating more fruits makes the teeth

to be free from stains because the

fibres helps to scrape off diets from

it. This makes plaques of the teeth to

be prevented. It also increase the

immunity of the body. After eating

fruits it is good to gargle the mouth

with clean water and swallow it. This

prevents fruit particles to not be

found in between and on the teeth.

This prevent fruit particles from

decomposition on the tongue that

can cause halitosis (bad breath). It

also prevents fermentation of sweet

fruits in the mouth by bacteria,

which when not prevented can

cause the formation of plaques on

the teeth, acid formation,which then

cause demineralization of teeth.

Which result to cavitation of the

teeth. And if untreated, it cause

infection from one tooth to another.

From the teeth infection, it migrates to the gum infection (gingivopathy). It is very important to keep the tongue, teeth, palate and the whole mouth clean. This prevents disease to occur to the mouth.

The whole human body also needs to be taking good care of (body hygiene). Because, when diseases are not treated in any part of the body, the pathogen(disease causing organism) can migrate from that part that is not treated to another part of the body that is not affected. This is possible by moving via the blood in the blood vessels, via the lymphatic fluids in the lymphatic vessels and through cavities in the body. For example, via(through) the peritoneal cavity(cavity inside the abdomen). Infection can also migrate from the cerebrospinal fluid, this is fluid that is present in the brain and spinal cord. This can cause infection to the brain and the spinal cord.

Teeth grinding can wear the teeth.

This should be prevented from

happening.

Food That Is Good For Healthy Gums,

Teeth, Tongue And Palate.

Citrus fruits such as oranges, lemon,

lime, tangerines and guavas is good

to prevent scurvy. Scurvy is gum

disease.

Eating of cooked green vegetables as soup is good. This is because of the presence of folium that helps in the formation of blood. This make the teeth, gums, palates and tongue to be well nourished. Thereby preventing toothache, gum pain, palate pain and tongue pain. When there is low blood level in the human body(anaemia) it makes the person to feel pain in the body. Nociceptor are pain receptors that makes the body to be aware of pain in the body. When there is pain in the mouth it is very uncomfortable.

When there is low blood

level(anaemia), the teeth will not be

strong. This is because the gums are

fatigue(weak). The root of the teeth

in the alveolar bone is not very firm.

When there is hard hit on the mouth

it can easily cause teeth removal. It

is good to have oral(mouth) hygiene

and eat balance diet. This makes a

healthy mouth to happen.

Drinking healthy milk is good for

healthy teeth. It contain calcium and

phosphorus that is good for a

healthy teeth.

Eating cooked fish and eating well

washed fruits is very good for

healthy gums, palate, tongue and

teeth.

Drinking of soy milk is also very good

for a healthy mouth. After eating

food it is good to gargle the mouth

with water and swallow it. It makes

food particles that remains in the

mouth after eating to be removed.

This makes halitosis (bad breath)

formation after eating to be

prevented.

Food that may result to harmful

effect to the body when the teeth is

not well taking good care of are

sugar, fruits that are sweet and

starch.

The food when left in the mouth,

bacteria ferment it and it makes

plaque(calculi, tooth caries) to occur.

There is acid formation, this cause

demineralization(break down) of the teeth to occur. Thereby causing cavity of the teeth to occur.

Prevention is good. This is by brushing the teeth with toothbrush and toothpaste. This removes particles of food that are left in the mouth after eating. Thereby, preventing tooth caries and tooth cavity formation.

Eating of ice can make the teeth to wear easily and cause fracture to the teeth.

Chewing of plastic and metals can also wear and fracture the teeth.

Eating acidic fruits and not gargling the mouth with water and swallow can cause the teeth to demineralize. Acidic fruits are lime, lemon and grape. Fruits that are sour in taste are acidic.

Food That Can Cause Tooth decay When The Mouth	Sugar	Starch	Sweet fruits	Sugar cane	Chocolate

h Is Not Was hed.					

TheTable Shows Food That Can Cause Tooth Decay When The Mouth Is Not Properly Washed After Eating Them.

Mouth Infection

Infection of the mouth occur as a result of the presence of pathogens (disease causing organisms). Pathogens are viruses, bacteria, fungi, protozoa and parasites.

Pathogens cause infection by exposure to the part of the body. Then there is adhesion to that region. They invade the area. There is colonization of that region. There is toxicity(poisoning) and there is tissue damage and diseases. This can happen from faeces contact to the mouth. Another part of the body can be affected and it may cause infection to the mouth. Because the microorganisms that cause such infection can through the blood flow

to the mouth and cause infection to
it.

Tape worm, vibro cholerae,
entameba histolytica and Escherichia
coli can enter the body from the
hands that have touched faeces, that
are not washed with soap and water.
The pathogens can affect the throat
and intestine. This can cause
anaemia (low blood level) and
diarrhoea (frequent stooling that is
soft and watery).

The cause of infections are virus,

bactere, fungi and other pathogens.

Diseases Of The Teeth

Hypocalcemia is when the calcium

level of the teeth is low. This result

to the reduction of the strength of

the teeth. The teeth can easily

demineralize in this situation. Also

the teeth can easily crack due to the

reduction in strength. It is important

for the person to eat food that has

calcium. Food such as milk and fish.

Abrasion can also occur. The

structure of the teeth is not normal.

Eating balanced diet in order to

prevent this from happening is good.

And also not allowing the teeth to

have any hard substance like stone

to be chewed. It can also cause the

structure of the tooth to not be in

proper shape and size.

Discolouration can occur to the teeth through bacteria infection, by cocoa tea. This can happen when the teeth is not properly washed with toothbrush and toothpaste after meal is eaten. Injury can also cause the teeth to be discolored.

When the teeth is not properly washed, it makes fermentation of the food particles to occur by bacteria. This can result to acid formation. This can lead to wearing (eroding) of the teeth.

The teeth root can be destroyed through infection. Oral hygiene is good to prevent this. This makes the gums to be healthy and also the teeth.

There can be malformations of the teeth. Anodontia is when there is no tooth that is formed. Hypodontia occurs when the teeth that is formed is not complete. When the teeth is more than normal number is known as hyperdontia. When the teeth in the mouth is few, it is known as oligodontia. When the teeth size is smaller than normal it is called microdontia and in the reverse it is called macrodontia. Diastema is gap formed between teeth. When there is malformation of the teeth is an indication of malnutrition. When there is lack of balanced diet it can lead to malformation of the teeth development. Also injury can cause it. Cancer can also cause it. Preventive measures should be made in order for it not to occur. Preventing cancer is by not eating carcinogenic substances. For example, food that has additives and colorants. Not exposing the body to radioactive radiation that can cause tumour formation. And by feeding on natural source food. Eating a lot of fruits is very good.

Diagnosis is done in the hospital by the use of blood test, MRI, PET scan and X-ray. This help to know the cause of the disease, it's therapy (treatment), prognosis (future result) and prevention.

It is good to take positive steps in order to live in a healthy body way. Making sure the systems are healthy. The cardiovascular system (system of the heart and the blood vessels), skeletal system (system of the skeleton),lymphatic system (system of the lymph nodes), pulmonary system (system of the lungs), reproductive system (system of organs of reproduction), endocrine system(system of the endocrine glands), nervous system (system of the neurons), muscular system

(system of the muscles), digestive

system (system of digestion),

exocrine system(system of the

integument), renal system (system

of the kidney), haematopoietic

system (system of the formation of

blood), urinary system (system of

the formation of urine and also

immune system (system of immunity

of the body against infections). It is

also important to prevent other

infections of the body parts, because

such can eventually affect the gums,

teeth, palate, tongue and the mouth

as a whole. There should be

prevention of lower respiratory

infections, HIV/AIDS, diarrhoea,

tuberculosis, malaria, measles,

pertussis, tetanus, meningitis,

syphilis, hepatitis B, poliomyelitis,

diphtheria, measles, tetanus,

hospital acquired infection and

disease.

Diarrhoea Infection

This can occur as a result of eating unwashed fruits that contain pathogens (disease causing microorganisms) and by bathing with water that is not clean. This can make pathogens(disease causing microorganisms) to enter into the body via(through) the anus. Thereby, causing infection to the intestine which result to diarrhoea. Diarrhoea should be prevented by washing fruits well before eating. Also food should be cooked properly before eating and if not yet eating it should be covered properly, in order to prevent microorganisms that may be in the air that can affect the food. Thereby causing infections. Drinking of clean water is important. This prevents infection of the body through water infection.

Respiratory Infections

This can occur in a dirty environment.
Pathogens that may be in the air can
be inhaled through the nose or when
the mouth is opened in such
environment, it can be affected. This
can cause the disease causing
microorganisms to pass from the
nose to the lungs and infect the lung.
For example, tuberculosis is bacteria
infection of lungs.

Malaria Infection

This occur as a result of plasmodium
parasite in the blood. It destroys the

red blood cells and this result to anaemia (low blood level in the body). This is transmitted by anopheles mosquitoes. This can be prevented by using mosquitoes net during sleeping. And if somebody is infected, such should go to the hospital the doctor is going to prescribe antimalarial drug for the patient. The therapy (treatment) will cure the disease. The proper dosage of the drug should be used.

Tetanus Infection

This is bacteria infection that is transmitted through cut that is made to the body, when the body is injured. This can be prevented by not using sharp objects to play. In the hospital, a medical doctor can administer tetanus vaccine to prevent the disease.

Hospital Acquired Infection

Infection of the body can occur in the hospital. The medical doctor can be infected by having the needle of a syringe that as been inserted into an infected person by a disease is unintentionally inserted into part of his or her body. This should be prevented. The medical doctor should discard used syringes. And the use of the same syringe from one patient to another should be prevented, because it can result to the transfer of infection from one patient to another. Hepatitis, Poliomyelitis, diphtheria and measles can be prevented by using the approximate vaccines in the hospital by the medical doctor

Insects

Insects such as lice can cause blood

to be sucked from the body. This

cause reduction of blood. This can

lead to anaemia (low blood level in

the body). This can be prevented by

fumigating the environment. And

also washing the head and hair

properly with water. This prevents

lice to be present on the hair and

therefore, preventing blood loss.

This eventually prevents gum and

teeth pain that can occur as a result

of low blood level (anaemia).

Washing the body well with soap

and water during bathing is good.

Steps To Be Taken That Is Beneficial

It is good to set alarm in the morning and in the night when to brush the teeth.

It is good to brush the teeth of little children by parents. This makes the teeth to be properly clean and healthy. It is also important to teach the children how to brush the teeth.

Brushing teeth while looking at the mirror make the person brushing his or teeth to be able to brush away diets and food particles from the teeth and tongue. Also looking at the mirror is good in order to examine properly the teeth, tongue, palate and other parts of the mouth effectively. This makes it possible to know if there is tooth decay or tooth cavity. And also to be able to make necessary steps in order to prevent infections.

Leaving the mouth for too long before cleaning it can cause infection to the mouth and other parts of the body.

Food that is too hot can cause burn to the gums. This can lead to exposure of the gums to infections.

Eating of iced food can lead to frostbite that can cause necrosis (death) of gum tissue. Gastric acid in the stomach can come to the mouth when there is regurgitation and cause the teeth to demineralize.

It is good to drink water in the morning in order to neutralize the acid in the stomach.

Don't use only toothbrush to clean the teeth. Use both toothbrush and toothpaste that has fluoride in it. Fluoride prevent tooth caries.

Don't use the fingers and toothpaste to clean the teeth. Don't use the fingers to replace the toothbrush it will not clean the teeth properly.

Don't use feathers to replace the toothbrush because it will not clean properly and it can cause infection to the mouth.

Parents should make sure their hands are clean, by washing it with soap and water before cleaning the mouth of their children.

Clean water should be used to gargle the mouth after cleaning of teeth with toothbrush and toothpaste that as fluoride in it. And also after the tongue as been brushed. The gargled water should be poured out and not swallowed. If swallowed can be harmful effect to the body.

Stay far from dirty environment when speaking. When talking in a dirty environment it can cause mouth infection to occur.

Don't use dirty handkerchief it can cause mouth infection.

Don't use dirty plate to eat, dirty plate can cause mouth infection.

Don't use dirty spoon to eat, dirty spoon can cause mouth infection.

Don't drink dirty water, dirty water can cause mouth infection.

Breathe with the nose and not with the mouth. When you breathe with the mouth it can make microorganisms that may be in the air to infect the mouth.

Close your mouth with handkerchief when coughing and go to the hospital to meet the medical doctor in order for him or her to prescribe drug for you to use for the cough to stop.

Take your bath frequently. This makes the lips to be clean.

Visiting the dentist is good, in order to have helpful information to keep the mouth clean.

Use tissue paper in the toilet and also soap and water. Wash hands well with soap and water after finishing using the toilet.

Avoid over brushing of the teeth. Over brushing of the teeth can lead to erosion of the teeth. It is good to brush in the morning after breakfast. This will help to remove food particles from the mouth that can cause infection. Also brushing of the teeth after dinner is good. This will make food particles to leave the mouth after dinner. This will prevent tooth decay and tooth cavitation.

Good oral hygiene is helpful. It prevent bad odour when speaking to people. It also prevent communicable disease from one person to another.

Over use of tetracycline drug can cause teeth discolouration.

Pulpitis: This is the inflammation of the tooth pulp. It can occur as a result of infection to the teeth. This cause pain to the teeth.

When there is inflammation of the alveolar bone, it is very uncomfortable. There is stress to open the mouth. There is pain in the cutting and chewing of food. There is difficulty to speak.

When there is abscess in the gums due to infection, it can lead to teeth infection. And when this is not properly treated it can lead to teeth removal.

It is good to properly take good care of the teeth in order to prevent pulp necrosis(pulp death).

When there is a lot of food particles between teeth it can cause teeth pain.

Pathogens can cause skin ulcer.

When ulcer occurs eating of acidic fruits such as lemon and lime can be very uncomfortable.

When there is infection to the muscles that functions for the mouth ability to chew. It makes chewing difficult or impossible.

Cancer of the palate can occur by eating food that are carcinogenic.

Cancer of the mucous membrane can occur by eating food that are carcinogenic.

Trans fat
Food additives
Food colorants

Synthetic drinks
Preservatives
Radioactive radiation

The above table shows what can

cause cancer.

| House hygiene |
| Environment sanitation |
| Bath regularly |
| Wearing neat clothes |

Eating of fruits
Eating of vegetables that is cooked
Eating natural food that is cooked

The above table shows what can

prevent cancer.

Brush in the morning after breakfast
Brush in the night after dinner
Look at the mirror when brushing as a guide
After brushing wash gargle with clean water and pour it out
Use mirror to examine teeth after

brushing
If there is dirt in some areas, wash again and make sure the mouth is very clean
Continue the procedure day and night, this makes oral hygiene to occur

Procedure to be taken to have oral

hygiene is shown in the table above.

General Mouth Care Procedures.

When there is dry mouth. It can be

as an indication of low water level in

the body. At that moment you can

drink enough water to make the

body to be hydrated. This makes the

dry mouth to stop and the mouth

will then be moist with saliva. Dry

mouth can make chewing and swallowing of to be difficult. This can be as a result of causing friction in the mouth. It can also cause carbohydrate food not to be properly digested, because it is amylase in the mouth that assist in starch digestion. Amylase in an enzyme that aid the digestion of starch food. When the body is well hydrated, this makes the salivary glands to produce a lot of saliva. This makes the amylase to be much for proper digestion of starch in the mouth.

Nociceptors makes the gums to feel pain when there is low level of blood in the body. It is good to eat cooked green vegetables, beef and liver in order to have enough blood. When there is bleeding gums due to deficiency of vitamin C. It is expected to eat food such as guava, orange and lemon that has vitamin C. This helps to treat the bleeding gums.

Hard toothbrush can also cause bleeding gums. It is good to use small head toothbrush that has soft bristles. This prevent bleeding gums when brushing the teeth.

It is good for parents to show children how to brush their teeth. And watch them brushing their teeth by them selves. Making sure that they do not swallow the liquid during brushing with fluoride toothpaste. It is expected of them to spit it out. The more the swallow the fluoride toothpaste, it can become toxic to the children. It is expected of them to spit it out and gargle the mouth with clean water and spit it out. The will prevent toxic occurrence to the children. They should also look at the mirror to see if there is any particles of food in the mouth. And if there is any it is expected for the children to brush again and make sure that the mouth is very clean and healthy.

It is good not to use metallic sharp objects on the teeth to remove food particles individually. It is expected to get medical advice from the medical doctor in order not to injure to teeth with the metallic sharp object. Metallic sharp objects can cause injury to the gums, tongues, palate and also the lips. Which can lead to low blood level in the body.

It good not to open the mouth to breath. This can make the mouth to be infected by disease causing microorganisms. It is good to use the nose to breathe. When the mouth is used to breathe, when infected by bacteria it can lead to mouth odor. When mouth odor occurs, it is good to brush the teeth with a soft bristles toothbrush and fluoride toothpaste. This will make the mouth free from mouth odor. And after then the nose should be used for breathing.

It is good to wash the face regularly.
This prevent disease causing
microorganisms not to infect the lips.
This makes the lips to be clean and
healthy.

It is very good to exercise the body.
This makes the mouth to be in
normal condition. Because when you
exercise the body obesity is
prevented. Diabetes mellitus is
prevented. This will prevent

unhealed bleeding gums. This will make the mouth to be in normal shape. This will make the lips not to be too big. It will make the lips to have normal shape.

Taking good care of the mouth prevent disease of the esophagus as a result of disease causing microorganisms from the mouth into the esophagus. Thereby preventing inflammation of the esophagus that can be caused due to pathogens

from the mouth into the esophagus.

Eating of green garden egg and

drinking the juice of lime is good to

prevent mouth infection. It is good

after eating garden egg and drinking

the juice of lime for you to gargle

your mouth with clean water and

swallow. This is because lime is

acidic it prevent pathogens from

infecting the mouth. Gargle your

mouth with clean water and swallow

because the acid of the lime, when it is too long in the mouth it can cause demineralized teeth. Gargling your mouth with clean water and swallowing it will prevent demineralized teeth.

Do not allow any injury(trauma) to the mouth. When there is breakage in the gums it can lead to access to bacteria to infect the gums. When you are riding bicycle wear the helmet. This prevent injury. When

you are on the motorcycle wear your

helmet this prevent injury. When

you are in the car buckle sit bet, this

prevent injury. When the mouth is

not injured this prevent disfigured

mouth. This makes the mouth to be

in the normal shape.

When there is knocked out tooth.

Quickly take it and put it back into

it's position. Don't allow it to dry by

leavind it aside. The moment it got

removed, putting it back into it's position can cause it to be healed. After placing it into it's position go and immediately see a medical doctor.

Teeth that is used to break hard but shell and opening package can make the teeth to break or get removed from it's position. This can lead to bleeding, which can cause anemia (low blood level)

It is good to have checkup from the

dentist. This prevent mouth diseases.

And you can have advice from the

dentist in order to have useful

information's that is beneficial to

keep the teeth clean and healthy.

This will make mouth infections to

be prevented. And if there is any

mouth disease so that there can be

treatment for it. This will make the

teeth, gums, tongue and the mouth

as a whole to have oral hygiene.

It is good for you to brush your teeth

very well. Brush different corners of

the mouth. This will not allow

plaque to form on the teeth. It is

good to leave the foam for a while in

the mouth before spitting it out. This

will prevent tooth caries. It is good

to gargle the mouth thoroughly with

clean water and spit it out.

Accumulation of toothpaste in the

body when swallowed can be toxic

to the body.

Don't smoke. Smoke can make the mouth to have cancer. There can be cancer of the tongue. There can be cancer of the palate. There can be cancer of the tonsil, there can be cancer of the lips and there can be cancer of the cheeks. Smoking can lead to inflammation of the tongue. It can lead to inflammation of the tonsil. It can lead to inflammation of the palate. It can lead to inflammation of the lips and it can lead to the inflammation of the inner surface of the cheeks. Smoking can lead to tooth decay. Smoking can cause teeth discoloration. Smoking can cause bad breath. Smoking can make the teeth not to have enough nutrient from the blood. This is because the blood when there is carbon monoxide from the smoke as free radical it will replace oxygen in the blood thereby making the gum to be less nourished. This can lead to weak gums. This can lead to weak teeth. And this can

result to teeth pain.

When the mouth is not properly

taken care of. It can lead to the

salivary glands infection. This can

make the salivary glands not the

secret saliva normally. This can make

food not to be well digested when it

is eaten and swallowed. The saliva

that is produced can be infected.

This can cause the food that is

swallowed to be infected. This can

lead to disease of the stomach and

the intestines.

It is good not to have self medication

to resolve tooth pain. It is good to go

and see the medical doctor when

there is tooth pain in order for any

adverse effect not to occur.